Strain

Grower

Date

Acquired

$

| Indica | Hybrid | Sativa |

☐ Flower ☐ Edible ☐ Concentrate

Symptoms Relieved

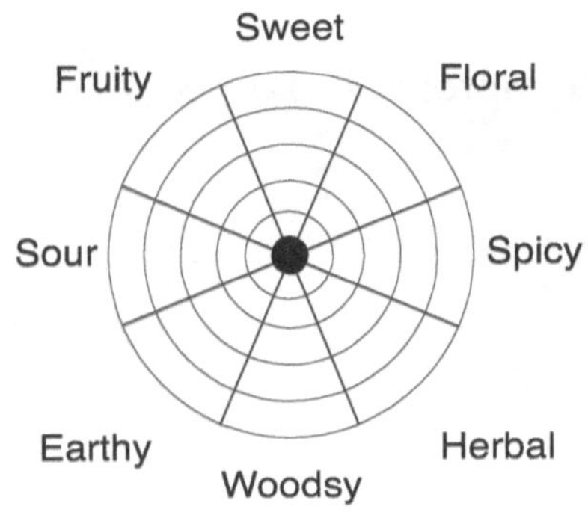

Notes

Effects	Strength
Peaceful	○ ○ ○ ○ ○
Sleepy	○ ○ ○ ○ ○
Pain Relief	○ ○ ○ ○ ○
Hungry	○ ○ ○ ○ ○
Uplifted	○ ○ ○ ○ ○
Creative	○ ○ ○ ○ ○

Ratings ☆ ☆ ☆ ☆ ☆

Strain

Grower

Date

Acquired

$

| Indica | Hybrid | Sativa |

☐ Flower ☐ Edible ☐ Concentrate

Symptoms Relieved

Sweet

Fruity

Floral

Sour

Spicy

Earthy

Herbal

Woodsy

Notes

Effects	Strength
Peaceful	○ ○ ○ ○ ○
Sleepy	○ ○ ○ ○ ○
Pain Relief	○ ○ ○ ○ ○
Hungry	○ ○ ○ ○ ○
Uplifted	○ ○ ○ ○ ○
Creative	○ ○ ○ ○ ○

Ratings ☆ ☆ ☆ ☆ ☆

As of this publishing, January 2019, the medical use of marijuana (cannabis) is legal in 33 states, the District of Columbia, the territories of Guam, Puerto Rico, the Northern Mariana Islands and the U.S. Virgin Islands; as long as you have a doctor's recommendation. Another 14 states have laws that limit THC content or allow for the use of the CBD component of cannabis.

It is up to the user of this notebook to determine if their locale has legalized or decriminalized the use of cannabis for recreational or medical use and the author/publisher of this notebook is not giving any legal advice on the matter.

ISBN: 9781794630406

Imprint: Independently published

Strain

Grower

Date

Acquired

$

| Indica | Hybrid | Sativa |

☐ Flower   ☐ Edible   ☐ Concentrate

Symptoms Relieved

Sweet
Fruity
Floral
Sour
Spicy
Earthy
Herbal
Woodsy

Notes

	Effects	Strength
Peaceful	○ ○ ○ ○ ○	
Sleepy	○ ○ ○ ○ ○	
Pain Relief	○ ○ ○ ○ ○	
Hungry	○ ○ ○ ○ ○	
Uplifted	○ ○ ○ ○ ○	
Creative	○ ○ ○ ○ ○	

Ratings ☆ ☆ ☆ ☆ ☆

Strain

Grower

Date

Acquired

$

| Indica | Hybrid | Sativa |

☐ Flower ☐ Edible ☐ Concentrate

Symptoms Relieved

Sweet
Fruity
Floral
Sour
Spicy
Earthy
Herbal
Woodsy

Notes

Effects	Strength
Peaceful	○ ○ ○ ○ ○
Sleepy	○ ○ ○ ○ ○
Pain Relief	○ ○ ○ ○ ○
Hungry	○ ○ ○ ○ ○
Uplifted	○ ○ ○ ○ ○
Creative	○ ○ ○ ○ ○

Ratings ☆ ☆ ☆ ☆ ☆

Strain

Grower

Date

Acquired

$

| Indica | Hybrid | Sativa |

☐ Flower   ☐ Edible   ☐ Concentrate

Symptoms Relieved

Sweet

Fruity

Floral

Sour

Spicy

Earthy

Herbal

Woodsy

Notes

| **Effects** | **Strength** |

Peaceful ○ ○ ○ ○ ○

Sleepy ○ ○ ○ ○ ○

Pain Relief ○ ○ ○ ○ ○

Hungry ○ ○ ○ ○ ○

Uplifted ○ ○ ○ ○ ○

Creative ○ ○ ○ ○ ○

Ratings ☆ ☆ ☆ ☆ ☆

Strain

Grower

Date

Acquired

$

| Indica | Hybrid | Sativa |

☐ Flower ☐ Edible ☐ Concentrate

Symptoms Relieved

Sweet
Fruity
Floral
Sour
Spicy
Earthy
Herbal
Woodsy

Notes

Effects	**Strength**
Peaceful	○ ○ ○ ○ ○
Sleepy	○ ○ ○ ○ ○
Pain Relief	○ ○ ○ ○ ○
Hungry	○ ○ ○ ○ ○
Uplifted	○ ○ ○ ○ ○
Creative	○ ○ ○ ○ ○

Ratings ☆ ☆ ☆ ☆ ☆

Strain

____

Grower _______________________ Date _______________

Acquired _______________________ $ _______________

| Indica | Hybrid | Sativa |

☐ Flower ☐ Edible ☐ Concentrate

Symptoms Relieved

____

____

____

____

Sweet
Fruity
Floral
Sour
Spicy
Earthy
Herbal
Woodsy

Notes

____

____

____

____

Effects	Strength				
Peaceful	○	○	○	○	○
Sleepy	○	○	○	○	○
Pain Relief	○	○	○	○	○
Hungry	○	○	○	○	○
Uplifted	○	○	○	○	○
Creative	○	○	○	○	○

Ratings ☆ ☆ ☆ ☆ ☆

Strain

Grower

Date

Acquired

$

| Indica | Hybrid | Sativa |

☐ Flower ☐ Edible ☐ Concentrate

Symptoms Relieved

Sweet
Fruity
Floral
Sour
Spicy
Earthy
Woodsy
Herbal

Notes

| Effects | Strength |

Peaceful ○ ○ ○ ○ ○

Sleepy ○ ○ ○ ○ ○

Pain Relief ○ ○ ○ ○ ○

Hungry ○ ○ ○ ○ ○

Uplifted ○ ○ ○ ○ ○

Creative ○ ○ ○ ○ ○

Ratings ☆ ☆ ☆ ☆ ☆

Strain

Grower

Date

Acquired

$

| Indica | Hybrid | Sativa |

☐ Flower ☐ Edible ☐ Concentrate

Symptoms Relieved

Sweet
Fruity   Floral
Sour   Spicy
Earthy   Herbal
Woodsy

Notes

Effects	Strength
Peaceful	○ ○ ○ ○ ○
Sleepy	○ ○ ○ ○ ○
Pain Relief	○ ○ ○ ○ ○
Hungry	○ ○ ○ ○ ○
Uplifted	○ ○ ○ ○ ○
Creative	○ ○ ○ ○ ○

Ratings ☆ ☆ ☆ ☆ ☆

Strain

Grower

Date

Acquired $

| Indica | Hybrid | Sativa |

☐ Flower   ☐ Edible   ☐ Concentrate

Symptoms Relieved

Sweet

Fruity   Floral

Sour   Spicy

Earthy   Herbal

Woodsy

Notes

| **Effects** | **Strength** |

Peaceful ○ ○ ○ ○ ○

Sleepy ○ ○ ○ ○ ○

Pain Relief ○ ○ ○ ○ ○

Hungry ○ ○ ○ ○ ○

Uplifted ○ ○ ○ ○ ○

Creative ○ ○ ○ ○ ○

Ratings ☆ ☆ ☆ ☆ ☆

Strain

Grower

Date

Acquired

$

| Indica | Hybrid | Sativa |

☐ Flower ☐ Edible ☐ Concentrate

Symptoms Relieved

Sweet
Fruity
Floral
Sour
Spicy
Earthy
Herbal
Woodsy

Notes

| Effects | Strength |

Peaceful ○ ○ ○ ○ ○

Sleepy ○ ○ ○ ○ ○

Pain Relief ○ ○ ○ ○ ○

Hungry ○ ○ ○ ○ ○

Uplifted ○ ○ ○ ○ ○

Creative ○ ○ ○ ○ ○

Ratings ☆ ☆ ☆ ☆ ☆

Strain

Grower

Date

Acquired

$

| Indica | Hybrid | Sativa |

☐ Flower   ☐ Edible   ☐ Concentrate

Symptoms Relieved

Sweet
Fruity
Floral
Sour
Spicy
Earthy
Herbal
Woodsy

Notes

| **Effects** | **Strength** |

Peaceful ○ ○ ○ ○ ○

Sleepy ○ ○ ○ ○ ○

Pain Relief ○ ○ ○ ○ ○

Hungry ○ ○ ○ ○ ○

Uplifted ○ ○ ○ ○ ○

Creative ○ ○ ○ ○ ○

Ratings ☆ ☆ ☆ ☆ ☆

Strain

Grower

Date

Acquired

$

| Indica | Hybrid | Sativa |

☐ Flower ☐ Edible ☐ Concentrate

Symptoms Relieved

Sweet

Fruity

Floral

Sour

Spicy

Earthy

Herbal

Woodsy

Notes

Effects	**Strength**
Peaceful	○ ○ ○ ○ ○
Sleepy	○ ○ ○ ○ ○
Pain Relief	○ ○ ○ ○ ○
Hungry	○ ○ ○ ○ ○
Uplifted	○ ○ ○ ○ ○
Creative	○ ○ ○ ○ ○

Ratings ☆ ☆ ☆ ☆ ☆

Strain

Grower

Date

Acquired

$

| Indica | Hybrid | Sativa |

☐ Flower ☐ Edible ☐ Concentrate

Symptoms Relieved

Sweet
Fruity
Floral
Sour
Spicy
Earthy
Herbal
Woodsy

Notes

Effects	**Strength**
Peaceful	○ ○ ○ ○ ○
Sleepy	○ ○ ○ ○ ○
Pain Relief	○ ○ ○ ○ ○
Hungry	○ ○ ○ ○ ○
Uplifted	○ ○ ○ ○ ○
Creative	○ ○ ○ ○ ○

Ratings ☆ ☆ ☆ ☆ ☆

Strain

Grower

Date

Acquired

$

| Indica | Hybrid | Sativa |

☐ Flower ☐ Edible ☐ Concentrate

Symptoms Relieved

Sweet
Fruity
Floral
Sour
Spicy
Earthy
Herbal
Woodsy

Notes

Effects	Strength
Peaceful	◯ ◯ ◯ ◯ ◯
Sleepy	◯ ◯ ◯ ◯ ◯
Pain Relief	◯ ◯ ◯ ◯ ◯
Hungry	◯ ◯ ◯ ◯ ◯
Uplifted	◯ ◯ ◯ ◯ ◯
Creative	◯ ◯ ◯ ◯ ◯

Ratings ☆ ☆ ☆ ☆ ☆

Strain

Grower

Date

Acquired

$

| Indica | Hybrid | Sativa |

☐ Flower ☐ Edible ☐ Concentrate

Symptoms Relieved

Notes

Effects	Strength
Peaceful	○ ○ ○ ○ ○
Sleepy	○ ○ ○ ○ ○
Pain Relief	○ ○ ○ ○ ○
Hungry	○ ○ ○ ○ ○
Uplifted	○ ○ ○ ○ ○
Creative	○ ○ ○ ○ ○

Ratings ☆ ☆ ☆ ☆ ☆

Strain

Grower

Date

Acquired

$

| Indica | Hybrid | Sativa |

☐ Flower ☐ Edible ☐ Concentrate

Symptoms Relieved

Sweet

Fruity

Floral

Sour

Spicy

Earthy

Herbal

Woodsy

Notes

| Effects | Strength |

Peaceful ○ ○ ○ ○ ○

Sleepy ○ ○ ○ ○ ○

Pain Relief ○ ○ ○ ○ ○

Hungry ○ ○ ○ ○ ○

Uplifted ○ ○ ○ ○ ○

Creative ○ ○ ○ ○ ○

Ratings ☆ ☆ ☆ ☆ ☆

Strain

Grower

Date

Acquired

$

| Indica | Hybrid | Sativa |

☐ Flower ☐ Edible ☐ Concentrate

Symptoms Relieved

Notes

Effects	Strength
Peaceful	○ ○ ○ ○ ○
Sleepy	○ ○ ○ ○ ○
Pain Relief	○ ○ ○ ○ ○
Hungry	○ ○ ○ ○ ○
Uplifted	○ ○ ○ ○ ○
Creative	○ ○ ○ ○ ○

Ratings ☆ ☆ ☆ ☆ ☆

Strain

____

Grower _______________________   Date _______

Acquired _______________________ $ _______

| Indica | Hybrid | Sativa |

☐ Flower   ☐ Edible   ☐ Concentrate

Symptoms Relieved

____

____

____

____

Notes

____

____

____

____

Effects	**Strength**				
Peaceful	○	○	○	○	○
Sleepy	○	○	○	○	○
Pain Relief	○	○	○	○	○
Hungry	○	○	○	○	○
Uplifted	○	○	○	○	○
Creative	○	○	○	○	○

Ratings ☆ ☆ ☆ ☆ ☆

Strain

Grower ___________________________   Date ___________

Acquired ___________________________ $ ___________

| Indica | Hybrid | Sativa |

☐ Flower ☐ Edible ☐ Concentrate

Symptoms Relieved

____

____

____

____

____

Notes

____

____

____

____

____

Effects	Strength				
Peaceful	○	○	○	○	○
Sleepy	○	○	○	○	○
Pain Relief	○	○	○	○	○
Hungry	○	○	○	○	○
Uplifted	○	○	○	○	○
Creative	○	○	○	○	○

Ratings ☆ ☆ ☆ ☆ ☆

Strain

Grower

Date

Acquired

$

| Indica | Hybrid | Sativa |

☐ Flower ☐ Edible ☐ Concentrate

Symptoms Relieved

Notes

Effects	Strength
Peaceful	○ ○ ○ ○ ○
Sleepy	○ ○ ○ ○ ○
Pain Relief	○ ○ ○ ○ ○
Hungry	○ ○ ○ ○ ○
Uplifted	○ ○ ○ ○ ○
Creative	○ ○ ○ ○ ○

Ratings ☆ ☆ ☆ ☆ ☆

Strain

Grower

Date

Acquired

$

Indica	Hybrid	Sativa

☐ Flower   ☐ Edible   ☐ Concentrate

Symptoms Relieved

Notes

Effects	Strength
Peaceful	○ ○ ○ ○ ○
Sleepy	○ ○ ○ ○ ○
Pain Relief	○ ○ ○ ○ ○
Hungry	○ ○ ○ ○ ○
Uplifted	○ ○ ○ ○ ○
Creative	○ ○ ○ ○ ○

Ratings ☆ ☆ ☆ ☆ ☆

Strain

Grower

Date

Acquired

$

| Indica | Hybrid | Sativa |

☐ Flower   ☐ Edible   ☐ Concentrate

Symptoms Relieved

Notes

Effects	**Strength**
Peaceful	○ ○ ○ ○ ○
Sleepy	○ ○ ○ ○ ○
Pain Relief	○ ○ ○ ○ ○
Hungry	○ ○ ○ ○ ○
Uplifted	○ ○ ○ ○ ○
Creative	○ ○ ○ ○ ○

Ratings ☆ ☆ ☆ ☆ ☆

Strain

Grower   Date

Acquired $

Indica	Hybrid	Sativa

☐ Flower   ☐ Edible   ☐ Concentrate

Symptoms Relieved

Sweet
Fruity
Floral
Sour
Spicy
Earthy
Herbal
Woodsy

Notes

Effects	Strength
Peaceful	○ ○ ○ ○ ○
Sleepy	○ ○ ○ ○ ○
Pain Relief	○ ○ ○ ○ ○
Hungry	○ ○ ○ ○ ○
Uplifted	○ ○ ○ ○ ○
Creative	○ ○ ○ ○ ○

Ratings ☆ ☆ ☆ ☆ ☆

Strain

Grower

Date

Acquired

$

| Indica | Hybrid | Sativa |

☐ Flower   ☐ Edible   ☐ Concentrate

Symptoms Relieved

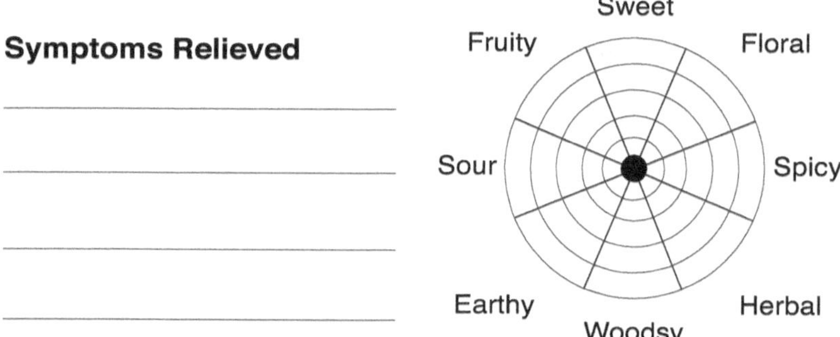

Notes

Effects	Strength
Peaceful	○ ○ ○ ○ ○
Sleepy	○ ○ ○ ○ ○
Pain Relief	○ ○ ○ ○ ○
Hungry	○ ○ ○ ○ ○
Uplifted	○ ○ ○ ○ ○
Creative	○ ○ ○ ○ ○

Ratings ☆ ☆ ☆ ☆ ☆

Strain

Grower

Date

Acquired

$

Indica	Hybrid	Sativa

☐ Flower ☐ Edible ☐ Concentrate

Symptoms Relieved

Sweet

Fruity

Floral

Sour

Spicy

Earthy

Herbal

Woodsy

Notes

Effects	**Strength**
Peaceful	○ ○ ○ ○ ○
Sleepy	○ ○ ○ ○ ○
Pain Relief	○ ○ ○ ○ ○
Hungry	○ ○ ○ ○ ○
Uplifted	○ ○ ○ ○ ○
Creative	○ ○ ○ ○ ○

Ratings ☆ ☆ ☆ ☆ ☆

Strain

Grower

Date

Acquired

$

| Indica | Hybrid | Sativa |

☐ Flower ☐ Edible ☐ Concentrate

Symptoms Relieved

Sweet
Fruity
Floral
Sour
Spicy
Earthy
Herbal
Woodsy

Notes

| **Effects** | **Strength** |

Peaceful	○ ○ ○ ○ ○
Sleepy	○ ○ ○ ○ ○
Pain Relief	○ ○ ○ ○ ○
Hungry	○ ○ ○ ○ ○
Uplifted	○ ○ ○ ○ ○
Creative	○ ○ ○ ○ ○

Ratings ☆ ☆ ☆ ☆ ☆

Strain

Grower

Date

Acquired

$

| Indica | Hybrid | Sativa |

☐ Flower   ☐ Edible   ☐ Concentrate

Symptoms Relieved

Notes

Effects	Strength
Peaceful	○ ○ ○ ○ ○
Sleepy	○ ○ ○ ○ ○
Pain Relief	○ ○ ○ ○ ○
Hungry	○ ○ ○ ○ ○
Uplifted	○ ○ ○ ○ ○
Creative	○ ○ ○ ○ ○

Ratings ☆ ☆ ☆ ☆ ☆

Strain

Grower ___________________ Date ___________

Acquired _________________ $ ___________

| Indica | Hybrid | Sativa |

☐ Flower ☐ Edible ☐ Concentrate

Symptoms Relieved

____

____

____

____

____

Notes

____

____

____

____

Effects	**Strength**
Peaceful	○ ○ ○ ○ ○
Sleepy	○ ○ ○ ○ ○
Pain Relief	○ ○ ○ ○ ○
Hungry	○ ○ ○ ○ ○
Uplifted	○ ○ ○ ○ ○
Creative	○ ○ ○ ○ ○

Ratings ☆ ☆ ☆ ☆ ☆

Strain

Grower

Date

Acquired

$

Indica	Hybrid	Sativa

☐ Flower ☐ Edible ☐ Concentrate

Symptoms Relieved

Sweet
Fruity
Floral
Sour
Spicy
Earthy
Herbal
Woodsy

Notes

Effects	Strength				
Peaceful	○	○	○	○	○
Sleepy	○	○	○	○	○
Pain Relief	○	○	○	○	○
Hungry	○	○	○	○	○
Uplifted	○	○	○	○	○
Creative	○	○	○	○	○

Ratings ☆ ☆ ☆ ☆ ☆

Strain

Grower _______________ Date _______

Acquired _______________ $ _______

| Indica | Hybrid | Sativa |

☐ Flower ☐ Edible ☐ Concentrate

Symptoms Relieved

____

____

____

____

Notes

____

____

____

____

Effects	**Strength**				
Peaceful	◯	◯	◯	◯	◯
Sleepy	◯	◯	◯	◯	◯
Pain Relief	◯	◯	◯	◯	◯
Hungry	◯	◯	◯	◯	◯
Uplifted	◯	◯	◯	◯	◯
Creative	◯	◯	◯	◯	◯

Ratings ☆ ☆ ☆ ☆ ☆

Strain

Grower   Date

Acquired $

Indica	Hybrid	Sativa

☐ Flower   ☐ Edible   ☐ Concentrate

Symptoms Relieved

Sweet
Fruity
Floral
Sour
Spicy
Earthy
Herbal
Woodsy

Notes

Effects	Strength
Peaceful	○ ○ ○ ○ ○
Sleepy	○ ○ ○ ○ ○
Pain Relief	○ ○ ○ ○ ○
Hungry	○ ○ ○ ○ ○
Uplifted	○ ○ ○ ○ ○
Creative	○ ○ ○ ○ ○

Ratings ☆ ☆ ☆ ☆ ☆

Strain

Grower

Date

Acquired

$

| Indica | Hybrid | Sativa |

[ ] Flower [ ] Edible [ ] Concentrate

Symptoms Relieved

Sweet

Fruity

Floral

Sour

Spicy

Earthy

Herbal

Woodsy

Notes

| **Effects** | **Strength** |

Peaceful ○ ○ ○ ○ ○

Sleepy ○ ○ ○ ○ ○

Pain Relief ○ ○ ○ ○ ○

Hungry ○ ○ ○ ○ ○

Uplifted ○ ○ ○ ○ ○

Creative ○ ○ ○ ○ ○

Ratings ☆ ☆ ☆ ☆ ☆

Strain

Grower

Date

Acquired

$

Indica   Hybrid   Sativa

☐ Flower   ☐ Edible   ☐ Concentrate

Symptoms Relieved

Sweet

Fruity   Floral

Sour   Spicy

Earthy   Herbal

Woodsy

Effects	Strength
Peaceful	○ ○ ○ ○ ○
Sleepy	○ ○ ○ ○ ○
Pain Relief	○ ○ ○ ○ ○
Hungry	○ ○ ○ ○ ○
Uplifted	○ ○ ○ ○ ○
Creative	○ ○ ○ ○ ○

Notes

Ratings ☆ ☆ ☆ ☆ ☆

Strain

Grower

Date

Acquired

$

| Indica | Hybrid | Sativa |

☐ Flower   ☐ Edible   ☐ Concentrate

Symptoms Relieved

Notes

| **Effects** | **Strength** |

Peaceful ○ ○ ○ ○ ○

Sleepy ○ ○ ○ ○ ○

Pain Relief ○ ○ ○ ○ ○

Hungry ○ ○ ○ ○ ○

Uplifted ○ ○ ○ ○ ○

Creative ○ ○ ○ ○ ○

Ratings ☆ ☆ ☆ ☆ ☆

Strain

Grower

Date

Acquired

$

| Indica | Hybrid | Sativa |

☐ Flower ☐ Edible ☐ Concentrate

Symptoms Relieved

Sweet

Fruity

Floral

Sour

Spicy

Earthy

Herbal

Woodsy

Notes

| **Effects** | **Strength** |

Peaceful ○ ○ ○ ○ ○

Sleepy ○ ○ ○ ○ ○

Pain Relief ○ ○ ○ ○ ○

Hungry ○ ○ ○ ○ ○

Uplifted ○ ○ ○ ○ ○

Creative ○ ○ ○ ○ ○

Ratings ☆ ☆ ☆ ☆ ☆

Strain

Grower

Date

Acquired

$

| Indica | Hybrid | Sativa |

☐ Flower ☐ Edible ☐ Concentrate

Symptoms Relieved

Notes

Effects	Strength
Peaceful	○ ○ ○ ○ ○
Sleepy	○ ○ ○ ○ ○
Pain Relief	○ ○ ○ ○ ○
Hungry	○ ○ ○ ○ ○
Uplifted	○ ○ ○ ○ ○
Creative	○ ○ ○ ○ ○

Ratings ☆ ☆ ☆ ☆ ☆

Strain

Grower ____________________   Date ____________

Acquired __________________ $ ____________

Indica	Hybrid	Sativa

☐ Flower   ☐ Edible   ☐ Concentrate

Symptoms Relieved

____

____

____

____

____

Notes

____

____

____

____

____

Effects	Strength				
Peaceful	○	○	○	○	○
Sleepy	○	○	○	○	○
Pain Relief	○	○	○	○	○
Hungry	○	○	○	○	○
Uplifted	○	○	○	○	○
Creative	○	○	○	○	○

Ratings ☆ ☆ ☆ ☆ ☆

Strain

Grower

Date

Acquired

$

| Indica | Hybrid | Sativa |

☐ Flower ☐ Edible ☐ Concentrate

Symptoms Relieved

Sweet

Fruity

Floral

Sour

Spicy

Earthy

Herbal

Woodsy

Notes

Effects	**Strength**
Peaceful	○ ○ ○ ○ ○
Sleepy	○ ○ ○ ○ ○
Pain Relief	○ ○ ○ ○ ○
Hungry	○ ○ ○ ○ ○
Uplifted	○ ○ ○ ○ ○
Creative	○ ○ ○ ○ ○

Ratings ☆ ☆ ☆ ☆ ☆

Strain

Grower

Date

Acquired

$

| Indica | Hybrid | Sativa |

☐ Flower   ☐ Edible   ☐ Concentrate

Symptoms Relieved

Sweet
Fruity
Floral
Sour
Spicy
Earthy
Herbal
Woodsy

Notes

Effects	**Strength**
Peaceful	○ ○ ○ ○ ○
Sleepy	○ ○ ○ ○ ○
Pain Relief	○ ○ ○ ○ ○
Hungry	○ ○ ○ ○ ○
Uplifted	○ ○ ○ ○ ○
Creative	○ ○ ○ ○ ○

Ratings ☆ ☆ ☆ ☆ ☆

Strain

Grower

Date

Acquired

$

| Indica | Hybrid | Sativa |

☐ Flower ☐ Edible ☐ Concentrate

Symptoms Relieved

Notes

| **Effects** | **Strength** |

Peaceful ○ ○ ○ ○ ○

Sleepy ○ ○ ○ ○ ○

Pain Relief ○ ○ ○ ○ ○

Hungry ○ ○ ○ ○ ○

Uplifted ○ ○ ○ ○ ○

Creative ○ ○ ○ ○ ○

Ratings ☆ ☆ ☆ ☆ ☆

Strain

Grower   Date

Acquired $

| Indica | Hybrid | Sativa |

☐ Flower   ☐ Edible   ☐ Concentrate

Symptoms Relieved

Sweet

Fruity   Floral

Sour   Spicy

Earthy   Herbal

Woodsy

Notes

Effects	Strength
Peaceful	◯ ◯ ◯ ◯ ◯
Sleepy	◯ ◯ ◯ ◯ ◯
Pain Relief	◯ ◯ ◯ ◯ ◯
Hungry	◯ ◯ ◯ ◯ ◯
Uplifted	◯ ◯ ◯ ◯ ◯
Creative	◯ ◯ ◯ ◯ ◯

Ratings ☆ ☆ ☆ ☆ ☆

Strain

Grower

Date

Acquired

$

| Indica | Hybrid | Sativa |

☐ Flower   ☐ Edible   ☐ Concentrate

Symptoms Relieved

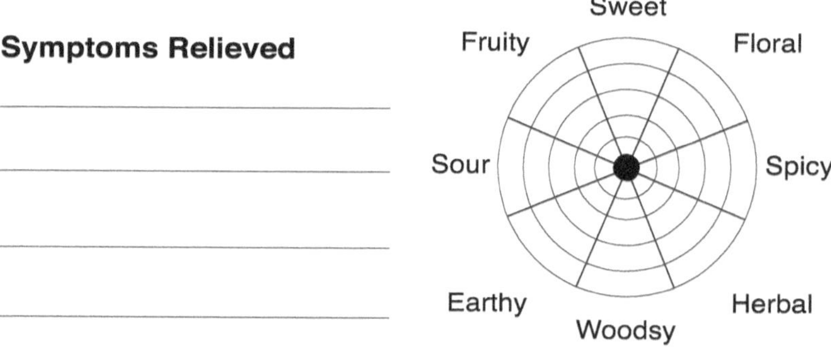

Notes

| Effects | Strength |

Peaceful ○ ○ ○ ○ ○

Sleepy ○ ○ ○ ○ ○

Pain Relief ○ ○ ○ ○ ○

Hungry ○ ○ ○ ○ ○

Uplifted ○ ○ ○ ○ ○

Creative ○ ○ ○ ○ ○

Ratings ☆ ☆ ☆ ☆ ☆

Strain

Grower

Date

Acquired

$

| Indica | Hybrid | Sativa |

☐ Flower ☐ Edible ☐ Concentrate

Symptoms Relieved

Notes

Effects	**Strength**
Peaceful	○ ○ ○ ○ ○
Sleepy	○ ○ ○ ○ ○
Pain Relief	○ ○ ○ ○ ○
Hungry	○ ○ ○ ○ ○
Uplifted	○ ○ ○ ○ ○
Creative	○ ○ ○ ○ ○

Ratings ☆ ☆ ☆ ☆ ☆

Strain

Grower   Date

Acquired $

Indica	Hybrid	Sativa

☐ Flower   ☐ Edible   ☐ Concentrate

Symptoms Relieved

____

____

____

____

____

Sweet
Fruity   Floral
Sour   Spicy
Earthy   Herbal
Woodsy

Notes

____

____

____

____

____

Effects	Strength				
Peaceful	○	○	○	○	○
Sleepy	○	○	○	○	○
Pain Relief	○	○	○	○	○
Hungry	○	○	○	○	○
Uplifted	○	○	○	○	○
Creative	○	○	○	○	○

Ratings ☆ ☆ ☆ ☆ ☆

Strain

Grower

Date

Acquired

$

| Indica | Hybrid | Sativa |

☐ Flower ☐ Edible ☐ Concentrate

Symptoms Relieved

Sweet

Fruity

Floral

Sour

Spicy

Earthy

Herbal

Woodsy

Notes

Effects	Strength
Peaceful	○ ○ ○ ○ ○
Sleepy	○ ○ ○ ○ ○
Pain Relief	○ ○ ○ ○ ○
Hungry	○ ○ ○ ○ ○
Uplifted	○ ○ ○ ○ ○
Creative	○ ○ ○ ○ ○

Ratings ☆ ☆ ☆ ☆ ☆

Strain

Grower

Date

Acquired

$

| Indica | Hybrid | Sativa |

☐ Flower   ☐ Edible   ☐ Concentrate

Symptoms Relieved

Sweet

Fruity

Floral

Sour

Spicy

Earthy

Herbal

Woodsy

Notes

Effects	**Strength**
Peaceful	◯ ◯ ◯ ◯ ◯
Sleepy	◯ ◯ ◯ ◯ ◯
Pain Relief	◯ ◯ ◯ ◯ ◯
Hungry	◯ ◯ ◯ ◯ ◯
Uplifted	◯ ◯ ◯ ◯ ◯
Creative	◯ ◯ ◯ ◯ ◯

Ratings ☆ ☆ ☆ ☆ ☆

Strain

Grower

Date

Acquired

$

| Indica | Hybrid | Sativa |

☐ Flower   ☐ Edible   ☐ Concentrate

Symptoms Relieved

Sweet
Fruity
Floral
Sour
Spicy
Earthy
Herbal
Woodsy

Notes

| Effects | Strength |

Peaceful ○ ○ ○ ○ ○

Sleepy ○ ○ ○ ○ ○

Pain Relief ○ ○ ○ ○ ○

Hungry ○ ○ ○ ○ ○

Uplifted ○ ○ ○ ○ ○

Creative ○ ○ ○ ○ ○

Ratings ☆ ☆ ☆ ☆ ☆

Strain

____

Grower _______________________ Date _______________

Acquired _______________________ $ _______________

| Indica | Hybrid | Sativa |

☐ Flower   ☐ Edible   ☐ Concentrate

Symptoms Relieved

____

____

____

____

Sweet
Fruity
Floral
Sour
Spicy
Earthy
Woodsy
Herbal

Notes

____

____

____

____

Effects	Strength
Peaceful	○ ○ ○ ○ ○
Sleepy	○ ○ ○ ○ ○
Pain Relief	○ ○ ○ ○ ○
Hungry	○ ○ ○ ○ ○
Uplifted	○ ○ ○ ○ ○
Creative	○ ○ ○ ○ ○

Ratings ☆ ☆ ☆ ☆ ☆

Strain

Grower

Date

Acquired

$

| Indica | Hybrid | Sativa |

☐ Flower ☐ Edible ☐ Concentrate

Symptoms Relieved

Sweet
Fruity
Floral
Sour
Spicy
Earthy
Herbal
Woodsy

Notes

Effects **Strength**

Peaceful ○ ○ ○ ○ ○

Sleepy ○ ○ ○ ○ ○

Pain Relief ○ ○ ○ ○ ○

Hungry ○ ○ ○ ○ ○

Uplifted ○ ○ ○ ○ ○

Creative ○ ○ ○ ○ ○

Ratings ☆ ☆ ☆ ☆ ☆

Strain

Grower

Date

Acquired

$

| Indica | Hybrid | Sativa |

☐ Flower   ☐ Edible   ☐ Concentrate

Symptoms Relieved

Sweet
Fruity
Floral
Sour
Spicy
Earthy
Herbal
Woodsy

Notes

Effects	Strength
Peaceful	○ ○ ○ ○ ○
Sleepy	○ ○ ○ ○ ○
Pain Relief	○ ○ ○ ○ ○
Hungry	○ ○ ○ ○ ○
Uplifted	○ ○ ○ ○ ○
Creative	○ ○ ○ ○ ○

Ratings ☆ ☆ ☆ ☆ ☆

Strain

Grower   Date

Acquired $

Indica	Hybrid	Sativa

☐ Flower   ☐ Edible   ☐ Concentrate

Symptoms Relieved

Sweet

Fruity   Floral

Sour   Spicy

Earthy   Herbal

Woodsy

Effects	Strength				
Peaceful	○	○	○	○	○
Sleepy	○	○	○	○	○
Pain Relief	○	○	○	○	○
Hungry	○	○	○	○	○
Uplifted	○	○	○	○	○
Creative	○	○	○	○	○

Notes

Ratings ☆ ☆ ☆ ☆ ☆

Strain

Grower

Date

Acquired

$

| Indica | Hybrid | Sativa |

☐ Flower   ☐ Edible   ☐ Concentrate

Symptoms Relieved

Sweet
Fruity
Floral
Sour
Spicy
Earthy
Herbal
Woodsy

Notes

| Effects | Strength |

Peaceful ○ ○ ○ ○ ○

Sleepy ○ ○ ○ ○ ○

Pain Relief ○ ○ ○ ○ ○

Hungry ○ ○ ○ ○ ○

Uplifted ○ ○ ○ ○ ○

Creative ○ ○ ○ ○ ○

Ratings ☆ ☆ ☆ ☆ ☆

Strain

Grower ___________________________ Date __________

Acquired ___________________________ $ __________

| Indica | Hybrid | Sativa |

☐ Flower   ☐ Edible   ☐ Concentrate

Symptoms Relieved

____

____

____

____

____

Sweet
Fruity
Floral
Sour
Spicy
Earthy
Herbal
Woodsy

Notes

____

____

____

____

Effects	Strength
Peaceful	○ ○ ○ ○ ○
Sleepy	○ ○ ○ ○ ○
Pain Relief	○ ○ ○ ○ ○
Hungry	○ ○ ○ ○ ○
Uplifted	○ ○ ○ ○ ○
Creative	○ ○ ○ ○ ○

Ratings ☆ ☆ ☆ ☆ ☆

Strain

Grower

Date

Acquired

$

| Indica | Hybrid | Sativa |

☐ Flower ☐ Edible ☐ Concentrate

Symptoms Relieved

Sweet

Fruity

Floral

Sour

Spicy

Earthy

Herbal

Woodsy

Notes

| **Effects** | **Strength** |

Peaceful ○ ○ ○ ○ ○

Sleepy ○ ○ ○ ○ ○

Pain Relief ○ ○ ○ ○ ○

Hungry ○ ○ ○ ○ ○

Uplifted ○ ○ ○ ○ ○

Creative ○ ○ ○ ○ ○

Ratings ☆ ☆ ☆ ☆ ☆

Strain

Grower   Date

Acquired $

| Indica | Hybrid | Sativa |

☐ Flower   ☐ Edible   ☐ Concentrate

Symptoms Relieved

Sweet
Fruity   Floral
Sour   Spicy
Earthy   Herbal
Woodsy

Notes

| **Effects** | **Strength** |

Peaceful ○ ○ ○ ○ ○

Sleepy ○ ○ ○ ○ ○

Pain Relief ○ ○ ○ ○ ○

Hungry ○ ○ ○ ○ ○

Uplifted ○ ○ ○ ○ ○

Creative ○ ○ ○ ○ ○

Ratings ☆ ☆ ☆ ☆ ☆

Strain

Grower

Date

Acquired

$

| Indica | Hybrid | Sativa |

☐ Flower ☐ Edible ☐ Concentrate

Symptoms Relieved

Sweet

Fruity

Floral

Sour

Spicy

Earthy

Herbal

Woodsy

Notes

Effects	**Strength**
Peaceful	○ ○ ○ ○ ○
Sleepy	○ ○ ○ ○ ○
Pain Relief	○ ○ ○ ○ ○
Hungry	○ ○ ○ ○ ○
Uplifted	○ ○ ○ ○ ○
Creative	○ ○ ○ ○ ○

Ratings ☆ ☆ ☆ ☆ ☆

Strain

Grower

Date

Acquired

$

| Indica | Hybrid | Sativa |

☐ Flower ☐ Edible ☐ Concentrate

Symptoms Relieved

Sweet
Fruity
Floral
Sour
Spicy
Earthy
Herbal
Woodsy

Notes

Effects	Strength
Peaceful	○ ○ ○ ○ ○
Sleepy	○ ○ ○ ○ ○
Pain Relief	○ ○ ○ ○ ○
Hungry	○ ○ ○ ○ ○
Uplifted	○ ○ ○ ○ ○
Creative	○ ○ ○ ○ ○

Ratings ☆ ☆ ☆ ☆ ☆

Strain

Grower

Date

Acquired

$

| Indica | Hybrid | Sativa |

☐ Flower ☐ Edible ☐ Concentrate

Symptoms Relieved

Sweet

Fruity

Floral

Sour

Spicy

Earthy

Herbal

Woodsy

Notes

Effects	Strength
Peaceful	○ ○ ○ ○ ○
Sleepy	○ ○ ○ ○ ○
Pain Relief	○ ○ ○ ○ ○
Hungry	○ ○ ○ ○ ○
Uplifted	○ ○ ○ ○ ○
Creative	○ ○ ○ ○ ○

Ratings ☆ ☆ ☆ ☆ ☆

Strain

Grower

Date

Acquired

$

Indica	Hybrid	Sativa

☐ Flower ☐ Edible ☐ Concentrate

Symptoms Relieved

Notes

Effects	**Strength**
Peaceful	○ ○ ○ ○ ○
Sleepy	○ ○ ○ ○ ○
Pain Relief	○ ○ ○ ○ ○
Hungry	○ ○ ○ ○ ○
Uplifted	○ ○ ○ ○ ○
Creative	○ ○ ○ ○ ○

Ratings ☆ ☆ ☆ ☆ ☆

Strain

Grower

Date

Acquired

$

| Indica | Hybrid | Sativa |

☐ Flower ☐ Edible ☐ Concentrate

Symptoms Relieved

Notes

Effects	**Strength**
Peaceful	○ ○ ○ ○ ○
Sleepy	○ ○ ○ ○ ○
Pain Relief	○ ○ ○ ○ ○
Hungry	○ ○ ○ ○ ○
Uplifted	○ ○ ○ ○ ○
Creative	○ ○ ○ ○ ○

Ratings ☆ ☆ ☆ ☆ ☆

Strain

Grower

Date

Acquired

$

| Indica | Hybrid | Sativa |

☐ Flower   ☐ Edible   ☐ Concentrate

Symptoms Relieved

Notes

Effects	**Strength**
Peaceful	○ ○ ○ ○ ○
Sleepy	○ ○ ○ ○ ○
Pain Relief	○ ○ ○ ○ ○
Hungry	○ ○ ○ ○ ○
Uplifted	○ ○ ○ ○ ○
Creative	○ ○ ○ ○ ○

Ratings ☆ ☆ ☆ ☆ ☆

Strain

Grower

Date

Acquired

$

Indica	Hybrid	Sativa

☐ Flower   ☐ Edible   ☐ Concentrate

Symptoms Relieved

Notes

Effects	Strength
Peaceful	○ ○ ○ ○ ○
Sleepy	○ ○ ○ ○ ○
Pain Relief	○ ○ ○ ○ ○
Hungry	○ ○ ○ ○ ○
Uplifted	○ ○ ○ ○ ○
Creative	○ ○ ○ ○ ○

Ratings ☆ ☆ ☆ ☆ ☆

Strain

Grower

Date

Acquired $

| Indica | Hybrid | Sativa |

☐ Flower   ☐ Edible   ☐ Concentrate

Symptoms Relieved

Notes

Effects	**Strength**
Peaceful	○ ○ ○ ○ ○
Sleepy	○ ○ ○ ○ ○
Pain Relief	○ ○ ○ ○ ○
Hungry	○ ○ ○ ○ ○
Uplifted	○ ○ ○ ○ ○
Creative	○ ○ ○ ○ ○

Ratings ☆ ☆ ☆ ☆ ☆

Strain

Grower

Date

Acquired

$

| Indica | Hybrid | Sativa |

☐ Flower ☐ Edible ☐ Concentrate

Symptoms Relieved

Notes

| **Effects** | **Strength** |

Peaceful ○ ○ ○ ○ ○

Sleepy ○ ○ ○ ○ ○

Pain Relief ○ ○ ○ ○ ○

Hungry ○ ○ ○ ○ ○

Uplifted ○ ○ ○ ○ ○

Creative ○ ○ ○ ○ ○

Ratings ☆ ☆ ☆ ☆ ☆

Strain

Grower

Date

Acquired

$

| Indica | Hybrid | Sativa |

☐ Flower ☐ Edible ☐ Concentrate

Symptoms Relieved

Notes

Effects	**Strength**
Peaceful	◯ ◯ ◯ ◯ ◯
Sleepy	◯ ◯ ◯ ◯ ◯
Pain Relief	◯ ◯ ◯ ◯ ◯
Hungry	◯ ◯ ◯ ◯ ◯
Uplifted	◯ ◯ ◯ ◯ ◯
Creative	◯ ◯ ◯ ◯ ◯

Ratings ☆ ☆ ☆ ☆ ☆

Strain

Grower

Date

Acquired

$

| Indica | Hybrid | Sativa |

☐ Flower ☐ Edible ☐ Concentrate

Symptoms Relieved

Sweet
Fruity
Floral
Sour
Spicy
Earthy
Herbal
Woodsy

Notes

Effects	Strength
Peaceful	○ ○ ○ ○ ○
Sleepy	○ ○ ○ ○ ○
Pain Relief	○ ○ ○ ○ ○
Hungry	○ ○ ○ ○ ○
Uplifted	○ ○ ○ ○ ○
Creative	○ ○ ○ ○ ○

Ratings ☆ ☆ ☆ ☆ ☆

Strain

Grower

Date

Acquired

$

| Indica | Hybrid | Sativa |

☐ Flower ☐ Edible ☐ Concentrate

Symptoms Relieved

Sweet
Fruity
Floral
Sour
Spicy
Earthy
Woodsy
Herbal

Notes

Effects	Strength
Peaceful	○ ○ ○ ○ ○
Sleepy	○ ○ ○ ○ ○
Pain Relief	○ ○ ○ ○ ○
Hungry	○ ○ ○ ○ ○
Uplifted	○ ○ ○ ○ ○
Creative	○ ○ ○ ○ ○

Ratings ☆ ☆ ☆ ☆ ☆

Strain

Grower   Date

Acquired $

Indica	Hybrid	Sativa

☐ Flower   ☐ Edible   ☐ Concentrate

Symptoms Relieved

____

____

____

____

____

Notes

____

____

____

____

Effects	Strength				
Peaceful	○	○	○	○	○
Sleepy	○	○	○	○	○
Pain Relief	○	○	○	○	○
Hungry	○	○	○	○	○
Uplifted	○	○	○	○	○
Creative	○	○	○	○	○

Ratings ☆ ☆ ☆ ☆ ☆

Strain

Grower

Date

Acquired

$

| Indica | Hybrid | Sativa |

☐ Flower ☐ Edible ☐ Concentrate

Symptoms Relieved

Sweet
Fruity · Floral
Sour · Spicy
Earthy · Herbal
Woodsy

Notes

	Effects	Strength
Peaceful	○ ○ ○ ○ ○
Sleepy	○ ○ ○ ○ ○
Pain Relief	○ ○ ○ ○ ○
Hungry	○ ○ ○ ○ ○
Uplifted	○ ○ ○ ○ ○
Creative	○ ○ ○ ○ ○

Ratings ☆ ☆ ☆ ☆ ☆

Strain

Grower

Date

Acquired

$

| Indica | Hybrid | Sativa |

☐ Flower   ☐ Edible   ☐ Concentrate

Symptoms Relieved

Sweet
Fruity
Floral
Sour
Spicy
Earthy
Herbal
Woodsy

Notes

Effects	**Strength**
Peaceful	○ ○ ○ ○ ○
Sleepy	○ ○ ○ ○ ○
Pain Relief	○ ○ ○ ○ ○
Hungry	○ ○ ○ ○ ○
Uplifted	○ ○ ○ ○ ○
Creative	○ ○ ○ ○ ○

Ratings ☆ ☆ ☆ ☆ ☆

Strain

Grower ___________________________

Date ___________

Acquired ___________________________ $ ___________

Indica	Hybrid	Sativa

☐ Flower ☐ Edible ☐ Concentrate

Symptoms Relieved

____

____

____

____

____

Sweet · Fruity · Floral · Sour · Spicy · Earthy · Woodsy · Herbal

Notes

____

____

____

____

Effects	Strength				
Peaceful	◯	◯	◯	◯	◯
Sleepy	◯	◯	◯	◯	◯
Pain Relief	◯	◯	◯	◯	◯
Hungry	◯	◯	◯	◯	◯
Uplifted	◯	◯	◯	◯	◯
Creative	◯	◯	◯	◯	◯

Ratings ☆ ☆ ☆ ☆ ☆

Strain

Grower

Date

Acquired

$

Indica	Hybrid	Sativa

☐ Flower ☐ Edible ☐ Concentrate

Symptoms Relieved

Sweet
Fruity
Floral
Sour
Spicy
Earthy
Herbal
Woodsy

Notes

Effects	**Strength**
Peaceful	○ ○ ○ ○ ○
Sleepy	○ ○ ○ ○ ○
Pain Relief	○ ○ ○ ○ ○
Hungry	○ ○ ○ ○ ○
Uplifted	○ ○ ○ ○ ○
Creative	○ ○ ○ ○ ○

Ratings ☆ ☆ ☆ ☆ ☆

Strain

Grower

Date

Acquired

$

Indica	Hybrid	Sativa

☐ Flower ☐ Edible ☐ Concentrate

Symptoms Relieved

Sweet
Fruity
Floral
Sour
Spicy
Earthy
Herbal
Woodsy

Notes

Effects	Strength				
Peaceful	○	○	○	○	○
Sleepy	○	○	○	○	○
Pain Relief	○	○	○	○	○
Hungry	○	○	○	○	○
Uplifted	○	○	○	○	○
Creative	○	○	○	○	○

Ratings ☆ ☆ ☆ ☆ ☆

Strain

Grower

Date

Acquired

$

| Indica | Hybrid | Sativa |

☐ Flower   ☐ Edible   ☐ Concentrate

Symptoms Relieved

Sweet
Fruity   Floral
Sour   Spicy
Earthy   Herbal
Woodsy

Notes

| **Effects** | **Strength** |

Peaceful ○ ○ ○ ○ ○

Sleepy ○ ○ ○ ○ ○

Pain Relief ○ ○ ○ ○ ○

Hungry ○ ○ ○ ○ ○

Uplifted ○ ○ ○ ○ ○

Creative ○ ○ ○ ○ ○

Ratings ☆ ☆ ☆ ☆ ☆

Strain

Grower

Date

Acquired

$

| Indica | Hybrid | Sativa |

☐ Flower ☐ Edible ☐ Concentrate

Symptoms Relieved

Sweet · Floral · Spicy · Herbal · Woodsy · Earthy · Sour · Fruity

Notes

Effects	**Strength**
Peaceful	○ ○ ○ ○ ○
Sleepy	○ ○ ○ ○ ○
Pain Relief	○ ○ ○ ○ ○
Hungry	○ ○ ○ ○ ○
Uplifted	○ ○ ○ ○ ○
Creative	○ ○ ○ ○ ○

Ratings ☆ ☆ ☆ ☆ ☆

Strain

Grower
Date

Acquired
$

| Indica | Hybrid | Sativa |

☐ Flower ☐ Edible ☐ Concentrate

Symptoms Relieved

Sweet
Fruity
Floral
Sour
Spicy
Earthy
Herbal
Woodsy

Notes

Effects	**Strength**
Peaceful	○ ○ ○ ○ ○
Sleepy	○ ○ ○ ○ ○
Pain Relief	○ ○ ○ ○ ○
Hungry	○ ○ ○ ○ ○
Uplifted	○ ○ ○ ○ ○
Creative	○ ○ ○ ○ ○

Ratings ☆ ☆ ☆ ☆ ☆

Strain

Grower

Date

Acquired

$

| Indica | Hybrid | Sativa |

☐ Flower ☐ Edible ☐ Concentrate

Symptoms Relieved

Notes

Effects	Strength
Peaceful	○ ○ ○ ○ ○
Sleepy	○ ○ ○ ○ ○
Pain Relief	○ ○ ○ ○ ○
Hungry	○ ○ ○ ○ ○
Uplifted	○ ○ ○ ○ ○
Creative	○ ○ ○ ○ ○

Ratings ☆ ☆ ☆ ☆ ☆

Strain

Grower

Date

Acquired

$

| Indica | Hybrid | Sativa |

☐ Flower   ☐ Edible   ☐ Concentrate

Symptoms Relieved

Sweet

Fruity

Floral

Sour

Spicy

Earthy

Herbal

Woodsy

Notes

| **Effects** | **Strength** |

Peaceful ○ ○ ○ ○ ○

Sleepy ○ ○ ○ ○ ○

Pain Relief ○ ○ ○ ○ ○

Hungry ○ ○ ○ ○ ○

Uplifted ○ ○ ○ ○ ○

Creative ○ ○ ○ ○ ○

Ratings ☆ ☆ ☆ ☆ ☆

Strain

____

Grower __________________________ Date __________

Acquired __________________________ $ __________

| Indica | Hybrid | Sativa |

☐ Flower   ☐ Edible   ☐ Concentrate

Symptoms Relieved

____

____

____

____

____

Notes

____

____

____

____

____

Effects	Strength
Peaceful	○ ○ ○ ○ ○
Sleepy	○ ○ ○ ○ ○
Pain Relief	○ ○ ○ ○ ○
Hungry	○ ○ ○ ○ ○
Uplifted	○ ○ ○ ○ ○
Creative	○ ○ ○ ○ ○

Ratings ☆ ☆ ☆ ☆ ☆

Strain

Grower

Date

Acquired

$

| Indica | Hybrid | Sativa |

☐ Flower ☐ Edible ☐ Concentrate

Symptoms Relieved

Notes

Effects	**Strength**
Peaceful	○ ○ ○ ○ ○
Sleepy	○ ○ ○ ○ ○
Pain Relief	○ ○ ○ ○ ○
Hungry	○ ○ ○ ○ ○
Uplifted	○ ○ ○ ○ ○
Creative	○ ○ ○ ○ ○

Ratings ☆ ☆ ☆ ☆ ☆

Strain

Grower

Date

Acquired

$

| Indica | Hybrid | Sativa |

☐ Flower   ☐ Edible   ☐ Concentrate

Symptoms Relieved

Notes

Effects	Strength
Peaceful	○ ○ ○ ○ ○
Sleepy	○ ○ ○ ○ ○
Pain Relief	○ ○ ○ ○ ○
Hungry	○ ○ ○ ○ ○
Uplifted	○ ○ ○ ○ ○
Creative	○ ○ ○ ○ ○

Ratings ☆ ☆ ☆ ☆ ☆

Strain

Grower   Date

Acquired $

| Indica | Hybrid | Sativa |

☐ Flower   ☐ Edible   ☐ Concentrate

Symptoms Relieved

Sweet

Fruity   Floral

Sour   Spicy

Earthy   Herbal

Woodsy

Notes

Effects	Strength
Peaceful	○ ○ ○ ○ ○
Sleepy	○ ○ ○ ○ ○
Pain Relief	○ ○ ○ ○ ○
Hungry	○ ○ ○ ○ ○
Uplifted	○ ○ ○ ○ ○
Creative	○ ○ ○ ○ ○

Ratings ☆ ☆ ☆ ☆ ☆

Strain

Grower

Acquired

Date

$

| Indica | Hybrid | Sativa |

☐ Flower ☐ Edible ☐ Concentrate

Symptoms Relieved

Sweet
Fruity
Floral
Sour
Spicy
Earthy
Woodsy
Herbal

Notes

Effects	Strength
Peaceful	○ ○ ○ ○ ○
Sleepy	○ ○ ○ ○ ○
Pain Relief	○ ○ ○ ○ ○
Hungry	○ ○ ○ ○ ○
Uplifted	○ ○ ○ ○ ○
Creative	○ ○ ○ ○ ○

Ratings ☆ ☆ ☆ ☆ ☆

Strain

Grower

Date

Acquired

$

| Indica | Hybrid | Sativa |

☐ Flower   ☐ Edible   ☐ Concentrate

Symptoms Relieved

Notes

Effects	Strength
Peaceful	○ ○ ○ ○ ○
Sleepy	○ ○ ○ ○ ○
Pain Relief	○ ○ ○ ○ ○
Hungry	○ ○ ○ ○ ○
Uplifted	○ ○ ○ ○ ○
Creative	○ ○ ○ ○ ○

Ratings ☆ ☆ ☆ ☆ ☆

Strain

Grower

Date

Acquired

$

| Indica | Hybrid | Sativa |

☐ Flower   ☐ Edible   ☐ Concentrate

Symptoms Relieved

Sweet

Fruity   Floral

Sour   Spicy

Earthy   Herbal

Woodsy

Notes

| **Effects** | **Strength** |

Peaceful ○ ○ ○ ○ ○

Sleepy ○ ○ ○ ○ ○

Pain Relief ○ ○ ○ ○ ○

Hungry ○ ○ ○ ○ ○

Uplifted ○ ○ ○ ○ ○

Creative ○ ○ ○ ○ ○

Ratings ☆ ☆ ☆ ☆ ☆

Strain

Grower

Date

Acquired

$

| Indica | Hybrid | Sativa |

☐ Flower   ☐ Edible   ☐ Concentrate

Symptoms Relieved

Sweet
Fruity
Floral
Sour
Spicy
Earthy
Herbal
Woodsy

Notes

Effects	**Strength**
Peaceful	○ ○ ○ ○ ○
Sleepy	○ ○ ○ ○ ○
Pain Relief	○ ○ ○ ○ ○
Hungry	○ ○ ○ ○ ○
Uplifted	○ ○ ○ ○ ○
Creative	○ ○ ○ ○ ○

Ratings ☆ ☆ ☆ ☆ ☆

Strain

Grower

Date

Acquired

$

| Indica | Hybrid | Sativa |

☐ Flower ☐ Edible ☐ Concentrate

Symptoms Relieved

Sweet
Fruity
Floral
Sour
Spicy
Earthy
Herbal
Woodsy

Notes

Effects	**Strength**
Peaceful	○ ○ ○ ○ ○
Sleepy	○ ○ ○ ○ ○
Pain Relief	○ ○ ○ ○ ○
Hungry	○ ○ ○ ○ ○
Uplifted	○ ○ ○ ○ ○
Creative	○ ○ ○ ○ ○

Ratings ☆ ☆ ☆ ☆ ☆

Strain

Grower   Date

Acquired $

| Indica | Hybrid | Sativa |

☐ Flower   ☐ Edible   ☐ Concentrate

Symptoms Relieved

Notes

Effects	Strength
Peaceful	○ ○ ○ ○ ○
Sleepy	○ ○ ○ ○ ○
Pain Relief	○ ○ ○ ○ ○
Hungry	○ ○ ○ ○ ○
Uplifted	○ ○ ○ ○ ○
Creative	○ ○ ○ ○ ○

Ratings ☆ ☆ ☆ ☆ ☆

Strain

Grower

Date

Acquired

$

| Indica | Hybrid | Sativa |

☐ Flower   ☐ Edible   ☐ Concentrate

Symptoms Relieved

Notes

Effects	Strength
Peaceful	○ ○ ○ ○ ○
Sleepy	○ ○ ○ ○ ○
Pain Relief	○ ○ ○ ○ ○
Hungry	○ ○ ○ ○ ○
Uplifted	○ ○ ○ ○ ○
Creative	○ ○ ○ ○ ○

Ratings ☆ ☆ ☆ ☆ ☆

Strain

Grower

Date

Acquired

$

| Indica | Hybrid | Sativa |

☐ Flower   ☐ Edible   ☐ Concentrate

Symptoms Relieved

Sweet

Fruity

Floral

Sour

Spicy

Earthy

Herbal

Woodsy

Notes

Effects	**Strength**
Peaceful	○ ○ ○ ○ ○
Sleepy	○ ○ ○ ○ ○
Pain Relief	○ ○ ○ ○ ○
Hungry	○ ○ ○ ○ ○
Uplifted	○ ○ ○ ○ ○
Creative	○ ○ ○ ○ ○

Ratings ☆ ☆ ☆ ☆ ☆

Strain

Grower ___________________ Date ___________

Acquired ___________________ $ ___________

| Indica | Hybrid | Sativa |

☐ Flower ☐ Edible ☐ Concentrate

Symptoms Relieved

____

____

____

____

____

Sweet · Fruity · Floral · Sour · Spicy · Earthy · Woodsy · Herbal

Notes

____

____

____

____

____

Effects	Strength				
Peaceful	○	○	○	○	○
Sleepy	○	○	○	○	○
Pain Relief	○	○	○	○	○
Hungry	○	○	○	○	○
Uplifted	○	○	○	○	○
Creative	○	○	○	○	○

Ratings ☆ ☆ ☆ ☆ ☆

Strain

Grower _______________   Date _______

Acquired _______________ $ _______

Indica	Hybrid	Sativa

☐ Flower   ☐ Edible   ☐ Concentrate

Symptoms Relieved

____

____

____

____

Notes

____

____

____

____

Effects	**Strength**
Peaceful	○ ○ ○ ○ ○
Sleepy	○ ○ ○ ○ ○
Pain Relief	○ ○ ○ ○ ○
Hungry	○ ○ ○ ○ ○
Uplifted	○ ○ ○ ○ ○
Creative	○ ○ ○ ○ ○

Ratings ☆ ☆ ☆ ☆ ☆

Strain

Grower

Date

Acquired

$

| Indica | Hybrid | Sativa |

☐ Flower   ☐ Edible   ☐ Concentrate

Symptoms Relieved

Sweet

Fruity

Floral

Sour

Spicy

Earthy

Herbal

Woodsy

Notes

	Effects	**Strength**
Peaceful	○ ○ ○ ○ ○
Sleepy	○ ○ ○ ○ ○
Pain Relief	○ ○ ○ ○ ○
Hungry	○ ○ ○ ○ ○
Uplifted	○ ○ ○ ○ ○
Creative	○ ○ ○ ○ ○

Ratings ☆ ☆ ☆ ☆ ☆

Strain

Grower

Date

Acquired

$

<table>
<tr><td>Indica</td><td>Hybrid</td><td>Sativa</td></tr>
</table>

☐ Flower ☐ Edible ☐ Concentrate

Symptoms Relieved

Sweet

Fruity

Floral

Sour

Spicy

Earthy

Herbal

Woodsy

Notes

Effects	Strength
Peaceful	○ ○ ○ ○ ○
Sleepy	○ ○ ○ ○ ○
Pain Relief	○ ○ ○ ○ ○
Hungry	○ ○ ○ ○ ○
Uplifted	○ ○ ○ ○ ○
Creative	○ ○ ○ ○ ○

Ratings ☆ ☆ ☆ ☆ ☆

Strain

Grower

Date

Acquired

$

| Indica | Hybrid | Sativa |

☐ Flower   ☐ Edible   ☐ Concentrate

Symptoms Relieved

Fruity Sweet Floral

Sour Spicy

Earthy Herbal

Woodsy

Notes

Effects	**Strength**
Peaceful	○ ○ ○ ○ ○
Sleepy	○ ○ ○ ○ ○
Pain Relief	○ ○ ○ ○ ○
Hungry	○ ○ ○ ○ ○
Uplifted	○ ○ ○ ○ ○
Creative	○ ○ ○ ○ ○

Ratings ☆ ☆ ☆ ☆ ☆

Strain

Grower

Date

Acquired

$

| Indica | Hybrid | Sativa |

☐ Flower ☐ Edible ☐ Concentrate

Symptoms Relieved

Notes

| **Effects** | **Strength** |

Peaceful ○ ○ ○ ○ ○

Sleepy ○ ○ ○ ○ ○

Pain Relief ○ ○ ○ ○ ○

Hungry ○ ○ ○ ○ ○

Uplifted ○ ○ ○ ○ ○

Creative ○ ○ ○ ○ ○

Ratings ☆ ☆ ☆ ☆ ☆

Strain

Grower

Date

Acquired

$

| Indica | Hybrid | Sativa |

☐ Flower   ☐ Edible   ☐ Concentrate

Symptoms Relieved

Sweet

Fruity

Floral

Sour

Spicy

Earthy

Herbal

Woodsy

Notes

| **Effects** | **Strength** |

Peaceful ○ ○ ○ ○ ○

Sleepy ○ ○ ○ ○ ○

Pain Relief ○ ○ ○ ○ ○

Hungry ○ ○ ○ ○ ○

Uplifted ○ ○ ○ ○ ○

Creative ○ ○ ○ ○ ○

Ratings ☆ ☆ ☆ ☆ ☆

Strain

Grower

Date

Acquired

$

<table>
<tr><td>Indica</td><td>Hybrid</td><td>Sativa</td></tr>
</table>

☐ Flower   ☐ Edible   ☐ Concentrate

Symptoms Relieved

Sweet
Fruity
Floral
Sour
Spicy
Earthy
Herbal
Woodsy

Notes

Effects	Strength
Peaceful	○ ○ ○ ○ ○
Sleepy	○ ○ ○ ○ ○
Pain Relief	○ ○ ○ ○ ○
Hungry	○ ○ ○ ○ ○
Uplifted	○ ○ ○ ○ ○
Creative	○ ○ ○ ○ ○

Ratings ☆ ☆ ☆ ☆ ☆

Strain

Grower

Date

Acquired

$

| Indica | Hybrid | Sativa |

☐ Flower ☐ Edible ☐ Concentrate

Symptoms Relieved

Sweet
Fruity
Floral
Sour
Spicy
Earthy
Herbal
Woodsy

Notes

Effects	Strength
Peaceful	○ ○ ○ ○ ○
Sleepy	○ ○ ○ ○ ○
Pain Relief	○ ○ ○ ○ ○
Hungry	○ ○ ○ ○ ○
Uplifted	○ ○ ○ ○ ○
Creative	○ ○ ○ ○ ○

Ratings ☆ ☆ ☆ ☆ ☆